Anti Aging Secret
Ultimate Guide to Look & Feel 10 Years Younger

Barbara Williams

Table of Contents

Introduction

The information provided in this book is about aging challenges and how to overcome them. It's about helping you make the right choices that will give you an opportunity to reflect on your health, lifestyle and ultimately the process of aging.

Gone are the days when reversing the aging process was an elusive dream. The aptitude to look younger than your age is not only a reality but achievable by anyone who is willing to make the right healthy choices. The beauty of it is that you don't have to spend a lot of money to look younger. This book reveals anti-aging secrets you've been seeking.

A wide range of factors can make anti-aging revolution a reality for those who are ready to take time, understand and assume the responsibility for their own well-being. Each chapter in this book will provide specific information on what adjustments you need to make in your life, not only live longer but to look younger as well.

From breaking your bad habits you already have and replacing it with the food and supplements you need to take, you are going to understand that aging is a phenomenon beyond human control. We are going to uncover solutions on how to counter its effects.

Unlike what most of us think, looking younger and living longer boils down to making very simple changes in your life. After reading this book, you will be surprised to know how thin the line between a youthful look and old age really is.

1: How to Slow Down the Aging Process

They say the more informed you are about inevitable changes, the easier it will be to handle them when they take place. While aging is inevitable, there are a few things you can do to slow down the process drastically, giving you more time to accomplish your goals in life. As a matter of fact, controlling your body deterioration boils down to making the right choices in how you live your life.

Here's are the 8 simple steps to slow down the aging process

1. Eat Right

You are what you eat, literally. According to health experts, eating at least five servings of fruits and vegetables for minerals and vitamins, as well as three servings of whole grains everyday helps your body repair damaged cells.

Avoid foods with additives and preservatives and ensure that your daily calories intake from fat doesn't exceed 35 percent. You can get 1 percent of your daily calories intake from milk or canola oil,

15 percent from foods rich in protein and the remaining calories from carbohydrates.

Foods with high protein content also help lower insulin level, guard against heart diseases and keep your weight in check. Avoid red meat which has been linked with clogged arteries and heart diseases. Eat fish, turkey or white eggs instead. Quit drinking and smoking too if you want to live longer.

2. *Embark on a Regular Exercise Regimen*

If you're serious about slowing down the aging process, you need to start an exercise program and stick to it. Countless studies so that exercise helps prevent loss of stamina, balance and bone density as we get older.

Health and fitness professionals recommend that you do a single set of 8 to 15 repetitions, using 8 to 10 exercises, 2 to 3 times every week for a full strength building program. Exercises make your tissues stronger, enabling them to handle stress and withstand trauma much better. Start slowly, moving from one exercise to another depending on your body's needs.

3. Take More Antioxidants

While free radicals are responsible for causing a number of age related diseases, they can be neutralized by antioxidants. Therefore, it goes without saying that your intake of antioxidants should remain at a reasonable level if you are in the quest to slow the aging process.

Antioxidants can be found in certain foods and supplements. Dark colored vegetables such as squash, carrots, tomatoes and spinach contain high levels of carotenoids while purple and blue berries are a great source for flavonoids.

Antioxidants found in food work through synergy and are often recommended over supplements, but if you want to go the supplements anyway, take at least 200 to 250 milligrams Vitamin C, 100 to 400 International Units (IU) of vitamin E and 6 to10 milligrams of carotenoid supplement.

4. Get Enough Sleep

Broken cells and tissues are repaired when you're in a deep soporific sleep. Also, growth hormones are produced during sleep. Research has it that if you have less than six to eight hours of sleep within a span of 24 hours, you have a greater risk of developing heart problems or experiencing stroke. As if that's not enough, your brain tends to deteriorate much faster.

Lack of sleep can make you restless and more susceptible to anger. People who do not get enough sleep are more prone to viral infections as well. Doctors recommend that you should at get at least eight hours of sleep a everyday for optimal health.

5. *Patch up Your Hormones*

Did you know that most patients who visit anti-aging doctors often complain about loss of energy, libido and stamina? These are the same symptoms that are associated with a decline in hormone levels.
Embarking on a hormone replacement therapy could be a great way to slow down the aging process, bearing in mind that the production of estrogen, testosterone, and progesterone decreases significantly when you hit 35. Medical practitioners are quick to note that a testosterone, estrogen, or progesterone prescription greatly improves a patient's well being.

6. Increase Your Brain Power

Develop a habit of reading books, magazines, newspapers and articles regularly. Fill and complete as many puzzles as you can. Know your hobbies and engage in them more often. When you use your brain, you not only make it sharper but increase its longevity as well.

Keep off artificial sweeteners; some studies have revealed they can cause brain's deterioration thanks to their excitotoxin effects. Basically, they overstimulate brain cells until they die, or it may cause diseases such as dementia or Alzheimer's.

7. *Protect Your Skin*

Skin is the biggest organ in the human body and also one of the most vulnerable. It's exposed to a number of harmful elements. To guard your skin against the harmful UV rays of the sun, wear a sunscreen when you're outdoors.

Add moisture to your skin by use of a natural moisturizer to protect the skin from breaking down. Apply a lotion made from essential oils and water formulations. Avoid alcohol based lotions as they may leave your skin with a dry feel.

Exfoliate regularly to unblock clogged pores and avoid chemicals that will deplete your skin and body. When you take good care of your skin, you will keep wrinkles and lines at bay thereby leaving the skin feeling soft and looking much younger.

8. *Be Happy*

Learn to appreciate the fact that you cannot change everything the way you wanted to be in life. Accept the fact that things will not always go as planned even if the plan was well calculated. Learn to develop positive thinking as well. When you learn to accept the things we cannot change, you end up living a happier, more fulfilled life.

Spend time with your family and volunteer for a worthy cause once in a while. Broaden your horizons, meet new friends and have some fun while you're still young. Meditate when you have time, and learn to forgive others as this helps you deal with stress and depression. Have a good laugh and remember to keep in touch with your close friends.

We all have one life to live so you should give it your best shot. While we can't run away from the fact that we will grow old, we don't have to live a short, unfulfilled life. With these simple steps to slow down the aging process, you can ensure you have more time on your hands to leave your name.

2: Best Anti-Aging Secrets Revealed

You've been there at one point or another in your life; that moment when you find yourself staring at the news anchor, your hairdresser or even your dentist and wondered, how do they manage to maintain such a youthful look, a well-toned body, great hair and flawless teeth not to mention a pore free complexion?

Defying age is not as hard. It's the simple things many of us ignore that make the biggest difference. Here are the best anti-aging secrets.

1. *Drink a Lot of Water*

Yes! I bet you've heard this over and over again and there are some good reasons to it. Drinking a lot of water is perhaps the easiest and the cheapest way to make sure you maintain a youthful and beautiful look. Water hydrates the skin, smooths out fine lines and moisture your skin for a radiant and healthy appearance. To derive maximum benefits, it's recommended that you drink at least 8 glasses of water everyday.

2. *Don't Take White Sugar*

Avoid processed sugar in your diet by all costs. Not only does white sugar speed up the aging process but leads to weakening of the collagen in your skin which eventually causes impulsive sagging and wrinkle formation. Use it to scrub your skin instead. You can slather a handful of white sugar all over your face and body to make your skin smooth and create a good canvas for makeup.

3. *Eat Spinach*

The health benefits of spinach are innumerable. Make spinach a healthy portion of your diet everyday as it helps keep cellulite at bay besides giving your skin a radiant look. This vegetable is also laded with a good dose of antioxidants that are essential for fighting wrinkles and fine lines on your face.

Throw a handful of spinach cuttings in your morning berry smoothie and you will have an incredible anti-aging breakfast in your hands.

4. *Take Supplements*

For most people, eating the recommended amount of vegetables, nutrient and fruits may be a daunting task. Thankfully, you can take multi-vitamin supplements to supply your body with the same nutrients provided by fruits and vegetables. You may consider taking particular types mineral supplements as well as calcium and iron to ensure optimum health on your body.

5. *Stop Using Makeup*

For women, use of makeup is not one of the best anti-aging secrets on the book. While there might be some truth that makeup makes you look younger, there are a couple of things you should know if you want to maintain a healthy, young and beautiful look.

Cream and powder foundations could be your worst enemy. As you age, the wrinkles around your mouth and eyes are unavoidable. Creams and moisturizers only decrease their appearance but don't eliminate them totally. As a matter of fact, your wrinkles will be more noticeable when your face is free of makeup. Ditch the makeup and you'll look younger instantly.

6. *Drink Red Wine*

Most people would be happy that drinking red wine is on the list of anti-aging secrets. According to research, drinking red wine reduces stress which has been sighted as one of the leading causes of aging. Also, red wine is full of antioxidants that are beneficial when it comes to slowing down the aging process. One or two glasses of wine is what you need on a daily basis; anything more than that becomes unhealthy.

7. *Use Topical Anti-Aging Creams*

There's a difference between makeup and topical anti-aging creams. While makeup doesn't fight aging, anti-aging creams do. The best anti-aging creams repair the aging process thanks to a Vitamin A derivative they contain. The Vitamin A derivative is known to boost collagen production and cell turnover.

Topical anti-aging creams unclog blocked pores, stimulate blood circulation, reduce oil, and acne formation which give you a smoother, brighter, and healthier appearance. Most of these creams are available over the counter but it's always advisable to seek advice from a dermatologist for the best product that matches your skin type.

8. *Fall in Love*

Falling in love is the greatest feeling in the world, so they say. Being in love is not a bad thing after all considering that it makes you glow from the inside out. Love is derived from tight family units in addition to warm and close relationships with other friends. Having a more fulfilling sex life goes a long way in reducing stress which by extension means a longer life.

9. *Have a Sensual Massage Once in a While*

Massage is known to have positive effects on the human body. When you move blocked energy through massage it makes you feel younger from inside out. Reflexology and deep tissue massages are particularly helpful in fighting aging.
If you don't have the money and time to hire a masseuse or visit a massage parlor, you can achieve the same benefits of massage by stretching, calming yourself and breathing deeply inside out for at least 20 minutes every day.

10. *Drink Tea and Coffee Quickly*

If you relish white flawless teeth, you need to check on the time spent drinking a cup of coffee or tea. If you sip tea or coffee for over an hour, you risk staining your teeth due to the coating and re-coating effect. This is the same for other staining liquids such as dark juices. A beautiful smile will not only make you look younger but bolsters you confidence as well; an important factor when it comes to living a longer and healthier life.

11. *Consider Fish Oil*

By now you know that anti-inflammatory foods are some of the best kept anti-aging secrets you'll ever come across. Fish oil has powerful anti-inflammatory properties that help in the growth of your hair and suppleness of your skin.

Take three 500 milligrams of omega 3 fish oil capsules in the morning and evening and your body will thank you for it. You can literally change your skin's appearance within a few weeks of taking fish oil.

Staying young makes you feel good about yourself and somehow changes your outlook on life. Knowing the fact that you are not going to die any time soon means more concentration on day to day activities which in turn brings more tangible achievements in life.

As you can see, you don't have to spend a lot of money to stay young and healthy as revealed by these simple and practical anti-aging secrets.

3: Anti-Aging Super Foods

What if someone told you certain foods can help turn back the hand of time and make you look younger? Well, the fact that you can look younger and live longer by eating certain kind of foods is not a mirage; it's actually true. There are certain foods that can bolster your health and reduce the impact that comes with aging.

Below is a comprehensive look at 8 super foods that will protect you against diseases, improve your vitality and ultimately prolong your life.

1. *Berries*

All berries from blueberries to raspberries, to cranberries to strawberries are full of antioxidants like flavonols and anthocynanins, which are known to promote cellular health and protect you against certain diseases. For instance anthocynanins present in blackberries can help reduce the risk of contracting cancer and diabetes.

Darker berries contain blue or black pigment which has a propensity of providing the best anti-aging benefits. They have the highest concentration of antioxidants. According to research, blueberries can even reduce neurological degeneration, enhance memory, reduce inflammation and keep the growth of cancer cells in check.

Berries are also a great source of vitamins, particularly vitamin C which is excellent for your skin. Moreover, vitamin C can help repair damaged tissues. It has also been associated with cancer prevention.

2. *Dark Chocolate*

Mostly, the effects of aging are seen on the skin. This is due to its exposure to ultra violet radiation. Eating or even drinking dark chocolate can reduce the effects of ultra violet radiation on your skin.

Studies have shown that Cocoa beans (from which chocolate is made) have the premier antioxidants than any other food. Eating dark chocolate can help increase blood circulation on the skin's surface, thereby boosting its capacity to retain moisture. This in turn reduces the appearance of wrinkles making you look much younger.

Not all chocolate help reduce aging. It's imperative to insist that it's only dark chocolate that has the greatest anti-aging benefits. Other forms of chocolate are more refined which takes away most antioxidant flavonols that are beneficial to the body.

3. *Beans*

Forget the fact that beans give you gas; they are good for your heart. Not only are they excellent dietary staples but is a great source of low fat protein particularly for those individual who don't eat meat.

Beans are laced with fibers which can help reduce cholesterol levels in the body. They have plenty of antioxidants and are chock full of essential vitamins and minerals such as vitamin B and iron as well as potassium.

As if that's not enough, some beans such as soy and kidney beans have protease inhibitors and genistein which are known to guard against cancer. Studies have revealed that individuals with high level of genistein in their bodies have the lowest risk of developing prostate and breast cancer.

4. *Fish*

Fish is one of the top anti-aging super foods and it's not a surprise that fish oil has been used often as a dietary supplement in the recent past. Fish and fish oil supplies the body with omega-3 fatty acids that can protect you against heart diseases. Omega-3 also reduces inflammation, lowers blood pressures and decreases the risk of arrhythmia.

People who eat fish often live longer. A study conducted among middle age men in America found that those who ate fish twice or thrice every week had a 40% lower mortality rate than those who didn't. The same study also revealed that men who had suffered heart attacks in the past had their mortality raised by 29% after eating fish twice every week.

Fish, unlike other meats is an excellent source of protein and contains low saturated fat. Doctors recommend that you eat fish or drink its oil supplement at least twice every week.

5. *Nuts*

Nuts contain high level of protein. All kinds of nuts are a great source of unsaturated fats. Just like cold-water fish, they are laded with omega 3 fatty acids which are good for your health.

Nuts are also a good source for vitamins and minerals such as potassium which helps reduce blood pressure. Furthermore, they contain vitamin

E which prevents cell damage and calcium for strong bones.

Another benefit derived from eating nuts is that they tend to fill you up without packing on pounds. This is due to the fact that up to 20% of nut's calorie content doesn't get absorbed by the body which makes them an excellent snack between meals.

6. *Whole Grains*

Eating whole grains is good for your digestive system. The high fiber content in whole grains will help your body flush out unwanted substances like fats and bad cholesterol. Fiber also helps keep your appetite in check besides controlling blood sugar.

The reason why whole grains are good anti-aging food is because grains such as oats, brown rice and whole bread are packed with important minerals and vitamins. Eating whole grains on a regular basis can lower your chances of experiencing stroke and heart disease.

Ensure that the grains you include in your diet are not refined as this strips away some vital minerals and vitamins which made them a good anti-aging super food in the first place.

7. *Garlic*

Garlic has been noted to add flavor to food. It has a number of anti-aging effects which include lowering blood pressure, cholesterol, and reducing inflammation.

Garlic also boosts the immune system and it's not surprising that it has been used to prevent and fight infections for centuries. Garlic has been associated with reducing the spread of cancer cells. You can use this super food to lower the risk getting intestinal, pancreatic, breast and stomach cancers as well.

8. *Avocado*

Avocados contain high volumes of monounsaturated fats, potassium, vitamin E and antioxidants. The vitamins and minerals contained in an avocado are known to lower cholesterol, blood pressure and improve skin health.

This anti-aging super food is also rich in foliate which reduces the risk of getting osteoporosis and heart attack. They also contain oleic acid, a monounsaturated fat that promotes formation of good cholesterol, and protection against blood clots.

All these anti-aging super foods are packed with nutrients and minerals that not only slow down the aging process but it helps keep away age related diseases. If you want to live longer, eat these foods on a regular basis and don't forget to exercise at least two to three times every week to combat aging effectively.

4: Secret to Look and Feel 10 Years Younger

How many times have you ever stared at that photo you took on the beach 10 years ago? You were young, your skin looked supple and you seemed to have all the fun in the world. How you wish you'd have such looks once again!

You may not go back in time but you can certainly change your looks to appear and feel 10 years younger or even better. All you need to do is put these measures outlined below to feel great and have that elusive younger look.

1. *Check Your Blood Pressure*

Anomalies in your blood pressure are one of the main reasons why you feel and look terribly old. The first step towards a youthful look starts by maintaining a healthy blood pressure. Check the blood pressure regularly to avert the risk of heart disease and other cardiovascular problems. For an improved blood circulation in your body, stay active.

2. *Cut out the Bad Habits*

Smoking and excessive drinking of alcohol make you appear much older than your age. Give up smoking for your lungs and respiratory system's sake. People who don't smoke or drink have a healthier skin tone. If you have been an addict for a long time, consider joining help groups or counseling centers to make your quest for a longer life a reality. Instead of alcohol, drink more water which has a lot of benefits to your body.

3. *Wrinkles beneath Your Eyes*

Apply eye cream to conceal the age-related circles and wrinkles beneath your eyes. According to health and fitness experts, you should consider using an eye cream that has been kept in the fridge. This lowers the cream's temperature for faster constriction of the blood vessels. This effectively reduces the puffiness and the circles under your eyes.

4. *Shape Your Eyebrows*

Long, unshaven eyebrows make you look much older. Get rid of any stray or any unnecessary long eyebrows as this will help improve your facial appearance. Besides shaping the eyebrows, you may consider shaving them off completely for a younger look.

Don't forget to keep your nails short and trimmed. Clean, well-trimmed nails give the reflection of a healthy body besides improving how you look.

5. *Change Your Wardrobe*

They say appearance is everything. As matter of fact, the first impression you give to the outside world has everything to do with the way you dress. As you get older, you might get out of touch with the trending dress codes and as a result appear older than you actually are. Get the right clothes that will make you look chic.

However, changing the way you dress doesn't mean wearing clothes that will attract unwanted attention. Just find the appropriate style and customize it to suit your taste and preference. This way, you will look and feel younger without doubt.

Start taking control of the undergarments you wear as well. The right underwear should give you a perky youthful appearance. This is especially true in women who want to get rid of those distracting panty lines that give an older look.

6. *Find the Right Hairstyle*

Long hair in men and women tend to give an impression of being too old or not having a sense of good grooming. As you get older, it becomes hard to maintain long hair.

To maintain a youthful look, trim the hair to a manageable level. Actually, shorter hair is better. Beware of cutting it too short in the name of looking young especially in women as this gives you a harsher, more masculine look.

7. *Whiten Your Teeth*

A bright warm smile always makes you look younger. However, you can smile from ear to ear if you have stained teeth. Chances are, if you've been drinking coffee or smoking for long time, your teeth is not as white as it used to be.

There is an array of products in the market today that can help whiten your teeth quickly. Conduct a research on such products and buy the one that suits you well.

8. *Modify Your Make Up*

While makeup may not help fight or slow down aging, it certainly does improve your appearance. However, you need to move with time. The kind of makeup you used 10 years ago doesn't necessarily have the same effects today. Modify your make up if you want to revamp your look to a much younger, fresher appearance. Pay a visit to the nearest mall and get yourself a makeover.

9. *Maintain a Healthy Weight*

The heavier you are, the older you appear. You need to shed off the extra pounds you've been carrying around if you want to improve the way you look. Lift some weight for strength building and to get your body well-toned. If you train at least two times a week, you will reduce your body fat by 3.7%.

Mild weight lifting for women also helps reduce abdominal fat and improves your waist line as well. Strength training boosts muscles responsible for burning calories stored by the body. When you have a lean body, you not only feel but look younger as well.

10. *Spend Time Outdoors More Often*

The fact that the sun can damage your skin's appearance and make you look older doesn't mean avoiding the sun by all means. You should spend more time outdoors as being exposed to nature may enhance your memory. When you view things in their natural setting, you're likely going to recall them the next time you see the same objects in photographs due to an improved memory. Go outdoors and enjoy the view as nature has a way of attracting your attention without requiring much thought.

11. *Take a Multivitamin*

According to research, a daily dose of multivitamins makes you healthier. Individuals who take multivitamins are 30 to 40 % healthier than individuals who get their vitamins from food only. Vitamins are crucial when it comes to hair growth and good skin health, two of the most important factors that make you look and feel young.

A lot for people look older than their age. Others feel old but that doesn't have to be that way. People will always try to look younger as they get older. With these easy tips, the look you've been yearning for is now within your reach.

5: Natural Home Remedies to Look Younger

Aging may be unavoidable, but aging in style is not. With everyone trying save money these days, you can still maintain a youthful look with effective, safe and cheap remedies that can be made at home with easy to find ingredients. The following is a listing of some home remedies you can use to counter aging effects for a younger and supple skin:

Lemon Juice Extract

Lemons contain vitamin C which is a strong antioxidant. Apart from its bleaching capabilities, lemon juice works wonders on freckles and age spots. Squeeze the juice out of the lemon, apply and leave it to sit on the skin for about 15 minutes then rinse it with warm water.

For better results mix one teaspoon of lemon juice to half teaspoon of milk cream and one teaspoon of egg white. Apply the mixture on the skin and rinse after 15 minutes with warm water.

Lemon juice mixed with honey is also very effective in dealing with aging skin because honey has a soothing effect. Just mix one teaspoon of lemon juice and honey then proceed to massage the mixture gently on your skin. Leave the mixture for 10 to 15 minutes before rinsing it off with warm water.

Coconut Milk

Coconut milk is chock full of vitamins and minerals that can help your skin look young and healthy. In addition, it has properties that can moisture your skin to keep it radiantly young, soft and supple.

Squeeze the milk out of grated coconut. Apply it on the skin and let it sit for around twenty minutes then rinse it off with warm water. Changes on your skin should be seen after a few weeks of daily use.

Papaya Mask

Papaya is famed for containing vitamin A which is good for your eyesight. Besides helping you with your eyes, you can use the fruit's mask to get rid of aging signs on your skin thanks to its strong antioxidant properties. Moreover, papaya contains an enzyme known as papain that can digest dead cells on the skin's surface to make it more elastic and firm.

To make the mask, cut a few pieces on an evenly ripe papaya and pound it into a smooth paste. Apply the paste on the skin and rinse it off after 15 minutes.

Rose Water

Rose water has a cleansing ability that can help get rid of dirt responsible for clogging skin pores. It can tighten the skin well due to its astringent properties. You can apply it under the eyes to reduce the age-related puffiness too.

Mix two teaspoons of rose water with three to four drops of glycerin and half a teaspoon of lemon juice. Apply the mixture on the skin using a clean cotton ball every night a few minutes before going to bed.

Alternatively, you can make a facial mask by mixing one teaspoon of rose water with one teaspoon of curd and one teaspoon of honey. Combine this mixture with pounded ripe banana and apply it on the face. Apply the mask and rinse off after 20 minutes with warm.

Cucumber Mixed with Curd

Cucumber can help reduce age related circles and puffiness under the eyes. In addition it can sooth your skin to keep it healthy. Curd has lactic acid which has the ability to exfoliate dead skin cells thereby helping rejuvenate your skin.

Mix two teaspoons of grated cucumber with half-cup of curd. Stir to mix and apply on the skin. Rinse the mixture off after 20 minutes with warm water. Use this mask twice every week for a few months and your skin will not only look young, but healthy as well.

Egg Whites

Touted as one of the best natural home remedies you can use to look younger, egg white will help mask the lines found under the eyes. You can also get rid of wrinkles and restore the skin's elasticity if you use the mask for a few months.

Beat one egg white until it's stiff and foamy. Apply the mask with a clean cloth or soft brush around the outer and inner eye areas and along the cheekbones as well. Leave it for 10 minutes. Spray the areas with warm water to remove the mask before drying with a cotton ball. Egg white is effective at reducing crow's feet as well.

Apple Cider Vinegar

Apple cider vinegar is very effective at exfoliating the skin externally. You can use the vinegar in two ways. First, you can apply it on the skin with a cotton ball few minutes before going to bed. Let the vinegar dry for around five minutes and rinse it off with warm water. Take extra caution when using apple cider vinegar for the first time as some people are allergic to it. If you're using it for the first time, you may consider diluting it with water.

Alternatively you can drink two teaspoons of organic cider vinegar with sixteen ounces of water all day long. Again, be extra careful as some individuals may have an allergic reaction to the acid contained in vinegar.

Cocoa Mixed with Honey, Heavy Cream and Oatmeal

Cocoa is one of the richest sources of polyphenol antioxidants which can help reverse aging by preventing oxidation caused by UV radiation. When combined with other natural moisturizers, cocoa can help rejuvenate your skin after damage from natural aging and pollution.

Mix quarter-cup of cocoa with three tablespoons of heavy cream and quarter-cup honey. Add three teaspoons of oatmeal powder to the mixture. Apply the thick mask on the skin and let it sit for about ten minutes before washing it off with warm water.

Olive Oil and Avocado Lotion

Avocados and olive oil are good for the skin especially dry skin which requires moisture and lipids to enhance natural barriers for a soft feel. The high levels of polyphenols in avocados and olive oil provides rich support for inner layers of the skin effectively giving it a smooth finish.

Take one tablespoon of avocado, mix it with two tablespoons of olive oil and half-cup of lemon juice. Stir until the ingredients are uniformly mixed.

Apply a thin layer of the lotion on the face and let it sit for the whole night. Rinse it off with warm water in the morning.

Natural home remedies are easy to make and most of all don't have any side effects associated with most anti-aging beauty products. However, just like with anything new, it's always advisable to test any home-made remedies before applying it on sensitive parts of the body, such as the face and beneath the eyes to see how your skin reacts to it. For instance, you can start by applying on the elbow before moving to other parts.

6: Anti-aging Secrets to Live Longer

Can you live to see your 100th birthday? Absolutely yes! In recent years, there has been ground breaking understanding on how the human body ages and what can be done to slow down of some of the worst impacts of aging. You can avoid age-related diseases, enhance your physical and brain power, not to mention your spiritual well-being if you abide by the secrets outlined below throughout your healthy and active life.

Take Care of Your DNA

As you get older, the split ends of your chromosomes (known to as telomeres) tend to get shorter. This in essence means that you become more susceptible to diseases. While most people think there is nothing they can do about this, a recent research suggests otherwise. In the maiden study, it was revealed that adjusting your lifestyle boosts production of enzymes that increase the length of telomeres. Thus, healthy living habits may slow down aging at the cellular level.

Be Meticulous

According to a research conducted recently, one of the best indicators of a long life is a meticulous and hardworking personality. The research found out that meticulous people are more persistent and pay more attention to every little detail of anything they embark on in life. It was found that these people go to great lengths to protect their health and make choices that lead to strong relationships and better careers.

Make Friends

Science states that having many friends might help you lead a longer life. A study conducted by Australian researches found out elderly people who are very social are less likely to die over a span of ten years compared to their counterparts who were less social. Close to a hundred and fifty other studies indicate that indeed there's a connection between having many friends and living longer. Someone once said, show me your friends and I will tell you who you are.

While friends may help you increase your longevity, you need to choose friends with healthy lifestyles. You're more likely going to become obese, if you hang around obese people. The same goes for other bad lifestyle habits such as smoking and drinking of alcohol. Have many friends but don't give into peer pressure; it might reduce your chances of living a long life.

Embrace Short Naps

Many people around the globe take naps when they have the time. There's enough evidence that napping could actually help you live longer. A survey that featured close to twenty four thousand participants puts forward that people who nap regularly are thirty seven percent less likely to die from heart disease than people who don't nap regularly. Scientists think that naps can help the heart's functionality by reducing stress hormones.

Make the Mediterranean Diet Part of Your Meal

The Mediterranean diet which includes whole grains, vegetables and olive oil as well as fish is good for your health and goes a long way in slowing down aging. Over fifty studies involving more than five hundred million people across the world reveal the remarkable benefits of this diet. The diet reduces the risk metabolic syndrome which includes a combination of increased blood sugar and pressure as well as obesity among other factors that elevate the risk of diabetes and heart disease.

Copy the Okinawan Eating Habits

The Okinawa people who reside in Japan had the longest life expectancy on the planet at some time. This was attributed to the fact that they mostly fed on traditional diet which included yellow and green vegetables that have low calorie content.

Most Okinawans are known to eat as much as eighty percent of the food on their plate. The life expectancy of the Okinawa may have dropped as the younger generation embraced other food but there's no doubt that traditional food can increase your life expectancy.

Get Married

Never mind that there's high rate of divorces but for those who manage to stick to it, marriage can be a good thing for your health. A number of studies show that people who are married have a propensity of outliving their unmarried counterparts. Researchers attribute this to the economic and social support that comes with marriage.

While sticking to a marriage might have a number of benefits, individuals who get divorced or widowed have a lower mortality rate than their counterparts who have never been married.

Manage Stress

Stress management is not only good for your heart but may actually reverse a heart disease. While you may not avoid stress given the hustles of this ever demanding life, there are a few viable options you can use to control it. Join a yoga class and develop the art of deep breathing besides learning to meditate once in a while.

Get in Touch With Your Spiritual Side

In a study conducted over a period of twelve years, it was discovered that people who were over sixty five years old and attended religious services had a higher level of vital immune system than those who didn't. It was evident that people who worship in unison have strong social bonds which contributed to their longevity.

Learn to Forgive

One of the best kept secret to live longer is the ability to forgive and let go. Forgiving those who offend you has surprising health benefits. Chronic anger is associated with reduced liver functionality, stroke, and cardiovascular diseases, among other ailments. Each time you forgive, you reduce apprehension, blood pressure and you can breathe more easily. All these factors combined will help you live a longer life.

Don't Lose Your Sense of Purpose

Find hobbies and activities that will keep you active in life. A team of Japanese researchers found that men without a strong sense of purpose were more likely to die from heart disease or stroke as compared to their counterparts who had a high sense of purpose. Another study indicates that when you have a strong sense of purpose, your chances of getting Alzheimer's disease are relatively low.

The clock starts ticking now. If you want to hit the 100th birthday and beyond, its time you implemented the above sighted anti-aging secrets. Use every trick on the book to remain as healthy as you can. Be aware of what might shorten your life and keep off the bad habit. Being conscious of how aging process work is the first step to understanding the doctrines that lie beneath anti-aging.

7: Anti-aging Nutritional Supplements

Aging is a natural, sometimes unpleasant fact. Why we get old is open to speculation even though molecular biologists attribute it to environmental factors such as smoking, stress and genetics. Irrespective of the reasons, many of us will do anything to stay young.

This being the case, it's not surprising to see why the sale of anti-aging supplements is poised to hit a staggering $ 291 billion by the year 2015. The biggest question then becomes, do these supplements really work? Are they worth your money and what is the science behind them?

To help you make better and informed decision, there are anti-aging supplements you may consider trying:

DHEA (Dehydroepiandrosterone)

DHEA is an adrenal hormone that is the antecedent for steroid hormones like estrogen and testosterone. It's the hormone responsible for maintaining a healthy skin tone, muscle mass and bone health.

The production of DHEA decreases as you advance in age in both men and women. DHEA supplements became widely used after a book dubbed DHEA and Aging was published by the New York Academy of Sciences. The supplement also gained popularity after it was established it can promote sexual libido and energy.

Coenzyme Q10 (CoQ10)

This is an enzyme produced by our bodies which is very vital for proper functioning of cells. It also helps in production of a molecule referred to as adenosine triphosphate or ATP. ATP is the fueling power being the energy-emitting center of a cell otherwise known as mitochondria.

As we advance in age, the production of Coenzyme decreases thereby interfering with the way body cells function. As a matter of fact, Parkinson's, cancer and diabetes patients have low levels of CoQ10 in their bodies.

According to researches, taking CoQ10 as a supplement can help lower the risk of heart disease. It may act as antioxidant, help in blood clotting and protect body cells against the effects of free radicals that cause the heart disease. In addition Coenzyme supplements may improve the overall health of diabetes patients by controlling blood sugar and cholesterol as well as blood pressure.

You can buy Coenzyme supplements in a number of forms including soft gel capsules.

Doctors recommend that you take CoQ10 in dosages of 30 to 300 milligrams for adults. There are usually no major side effects by using Coenzyme apart from occasional upset stomach. However, it's always advisable to consult a physician if you want to take the supplement when under medication.

Aspirin

Aspirin is known to take headaches away, reduce low grade fevers and relive minor pain. However for those with heart conditions, a low dosage of aspirin can help increase blood flow. A study carried in recent past showed that men who took aspirin on a daily basis didn't have to go through surgery to repair blocked blood vessels.

Aspirin may also help protect you against colon cancer. A study suggests that people who take aspirin more than sixteen times every month have a fifty percent lower chance of developing colon cancer because the tiny drug reduces the development of polyps usually associated with colon cancer.

However, it's important to mention that aspirin doesn't work for everyone. The reactions from men who use aspirin are different from women who use the same drug. Furthermore too much aspirin can cause stomach problems.

Carnitine

Carnitine is produced in the kidneys and liver. It's stored in the heart, brain, and muscles as well the sperm content. This is the nutrient that helps our bodies convert fat into energy. Carnitine pills are used by people whose bodies don't produce enough of the nutrient due to one reason or the other.

Some of the benefits derived from taking carnitine supplement include lowering the symptoms associated with Angina, a medical condition that causes extreme chest pains due to the lack of sufficient blood to the heart.

Acetyl-L-Carnitine has been hailed as having the ability to treat Alzheimer's disease. This is because this anti-aging nutritional supplement enhances memory. Carnitine is also used to relieve depression commonly associated dementia and senility. A number of studies suggest that L-carnitine supplements might increase sperm count in men.

Doctors recommend that you use carnitine depending on the ailment you're treating. The usual dose is between one to three grams per day. Individuals suffering from heart disease should use a dosage of 600 to 1200 milligrams three times per day. Other common dosages include:

- 1.5 to 2 grams per day for Angina and heart failure

- 2 to 4 grams per day for peripheral vascular disease

- 3 grams per day for diabetic neuropathy

- 300 to 100 milligrams 3 times daily for male infertility

- 500 to 100 milligrams 3 to 4 times per day for chronic fatigue syndrome

Fish Oil

Fish oil supplements contain fatty acids omega-3. Besides keeping the heart healthy, omega-3 reduces the overall risk of untimely death from coronary heart disease. Studies also show that fish oil helps lower triglyceride which is associated with cholesterol.

Old people use fish oil to keep the effects of age-related macular degeneration and glaucoma in check. Our bodies don't produce omega-3 fatty acids, thus taking fish oil supplement is imperative. Omega-3 also helps reduce pain and swelling in addition to ease blood clotting.

Beware of taking too much fish oil as excessive amounts may cause the blood to thin which in turn increases the chances of bleeding. Taking too much fish oil supplements may also harm your immune system hence reducing your body's ability to counter diseases. Fish oil can also hamper the effectiveness of birth control pills.

Fish oil supplement is found in soft get capsules. The recommended dosage is pegged at 1 to 4 grams of fish oil on a daily basis if you're seeking to lower high triglyceride levels. To fight high blood pressure, take 4 grams of fish oil supplement everyday. Fish oil can also help get rid of depression if taken in a dosage of 9.6 grams daily. Please remember that anti-aging supplements do not and should not be used as a replacement for conventional drugs.

Most anti-aging supplements work by restricting calories which is one of the rules of slowing down aging. Some supplements are available over the counter but it's always a good idea to consult a professional for advice on the best supplements available.

Conclusion

If you do not have a particular background on natural avenues to help you look and feel younger, this book presents all aspects of countering aging process in the most natural and inexpensive manner. There is no magical bullet to prevent aging, but there are certain things we can do to slow down the process.

However, to ensure that your goal is achieved, you need to be equipped with the right knowledge which is why this book was written.After reading the anti-aging secrets and tips provided in this book, you are now certainly on the right path to a long life. It must be emphasized that reading the book over and over again is not enough. You need to exercise what you've learned into action.

Some of the anti-aging tips discussed in this book may not provide instant results so you have to patient. The world is changing really fast and so are the anti-aging concepts. The information revealed here should be reviewed regularly to be in tandem with the latest anti-aging secrets to ensure that your quest to look and feel young is always up to date.

www.ingramcontent.com/pod-product-compliance
Lightning Source LLC
Chambersburg PA
CBHW071128280526
45787CB00003B/1217